SURVIVAL LESSONS

also by ALICE HOFFMAN

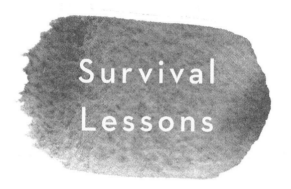

Survival
Lessons

ALICE HOFFMAN

ALGONQUIN BOOKS
OF CHAPEL HILL

2013

Published by
ALGONQUIN BOOKS OF CHAPEL HILL
Post Office Box 2225
Chapel Hill, North Carolina 27515-2225

a division of
WORKMAN PUBLISHING
225 Varick Street
New York, New York 10014

Library of Congress Cataloging-in-Publication Data is available.

Library of Congress Cataloging-in-Publication Data
Hoffman, Alice.
Survival lessons / Alice Hoffman.—First edition.
pages cm
ISBN 978-1-61620-314-6
1. Breast—Cancer—Patients—Psychological aspects.
2. Cancer—Patients—Attitudes.   3. Self-care, Health.
4. Hoffman, Alice—Health.   I. Title.
RC280.B8H628 2013
616.99'449—dc23   2013012811

10 9 8 7 6 5 4 3 2

When I found the lump I was convinced I had imagined it. These things didn't happen to me.

True, bad things happened around me. My mother was undergoing treatment for breast cancer. My sister-in-law had just lost her battle with brain cancer. Several relatives and friends were seriously ill. But, still, these things didn't happen to *me*. I was not someone who got cancer. In fact, I was the person who sat by bedsides, accompanied friends to doctor's appointments, researched family members' diseases until I became an expert, went to meetings with lawyers when divorce was the only option, found therapists for depressed teen-agers, bought plots at cemeteries, arranged funerals, babysat children and pets.

But as it turned out, I was also the one with cancer.

I did my best to pretend it wasn't so. I was busy after all, the mother of two young sons, caring for my ill mother, involved in my writing. My most recent novel, *Here on Earth,* had been chosen as an Oprah's Book Club selection; an earlier novel, *Practical Magic,* was being filmed in California with Sandra Bullock and Nicole Kidman. I didn't have time to be ill.

Now I know you can't run away by ignoring the truth. Truth follows you; it comes in through open windows and drifts under doors. I went for a biopsy, convinced I was fine. Days later my doctor phoned me and said, *Alice, I'm sorry.* Then I knew. Good fortune and bad luck are always tied together with invisible, unbreakable thread. It happens to everyone, in one way or another, sooner or later. The loss of a loved one, a divorce, heartbreak, a child set on the wrong path, a bad diagnosis. When it comes to sorrow, no one is immune.

I've always believed there is a very thin line that separates readers and writers. You make a leap over that line when there's a book you want to read and you can't find it and you have to write it yourself. All the while I was in treatment I was looking for a guidebook. I needed help in my new situation. I needed to know how people survived trauma.

It took all this time for me to figure out what I would have most wanted to hear when I was newly diagnosed, when I lost the people I loved, when I was deeply disappointed in myself and the turns my life had taken. In many ways I wrote this book to remind myself of the beauty of life, something that's all too easy to overlook during the crisis of illness or loss. There were many times when I forgot about roses and starry nights. I forgot that our lives are made up of equal parts sorrow and joy, and that it is impossible to have one without the other. This is what makes us human. This is why our world is so precious. I wrote to remind myself that in the darkest hour the roses still bloom, the stars still come out at night. And to remind myself that, despite everything that was happening to me, there were still choices I could make.

Fifteen years after being diagnosed with cancer, I've become something I never imagined I'd be. I'm a survivor.

We all experience trauma and we all take a very personal path to healing on our own terms. But we're also alike in what we need most. Love really is the answer. I received so many gifts from friends and strangers during my times of loss. I hope this book can be my gift to you.

Alice Hoffman

There is always a before and an after.
My advice, travel light.
Choose only what you need most
to see you through.

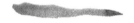

SURVIVAL LESSONS

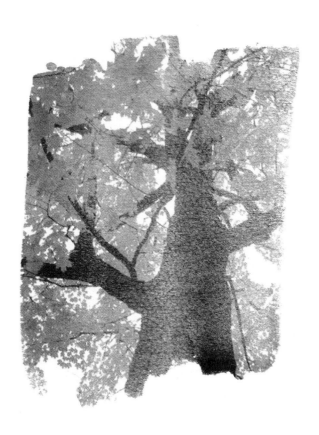

Choose
Your
Heroes

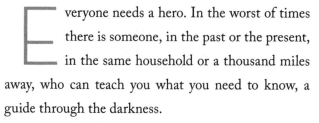

E veryone needs a hero. In the worst of times there is someone, in the past or the present, in the same household or a thousand miles away, who can teach you what you need to know, a guide through the darkness.

As a girl, I was obsessed with Anne Frank. She was young and a writer and Jewish, but most importantly, she was an optimist, able to keep her spirit strong even in the most brutal of times. She was my first hero, and I think I chose well. At the Anne Frank House in Amsterdam I'm always thrilled to see crowds of teenagers among the visitors waiting in line, all of them looking up to Anne Frank as I did, with awe and admiration. She wanted her life so much. She wanted to grow up and experience everything. She, along with her sister, did not survive the Bergen-Belson concentration camp, but her words, written into a checked autograph

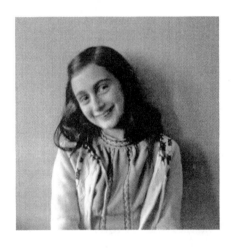

I don't think of all the misery,
but of the beauty that still remains.

—Anne Frank

book when she was hidden in an attic in Amsterdam, live on for us.

It's a wonder I haven't abandoned all my ideals, they seem so absurd and impractical. Yet I still believe, in spite of everything, that people are truly good at heart.

Anne Frank's passionate ability to see beauty in a cruel world is nothing less than astounding. Though she belongs to the past, she is the person I still look to for faith in the future.

It is difficult to measure a personal tragedy. How much bad fortune does it take to destroy a person? How much strength must someone possess in order to survive against the odds? In my house, my mother took to her bed when my father left her. She was in shock. I was eight years old and I didn't meet anyone else whose parents divorced until I was in college. Times were different then. A broken marriage was a stigma, a mark of real failure, a secret to hide away. For many it's still that way, an emotional earthquake.

My mother was a rebel, beautiful and lazy and brilliant. She thought she knew where her life was heading until the rug, which hadn't been vacuumed in months, was pulled out from under her. She completely fell apart. I slept on the floor of her room for several weeks because she was afraid to be alone.

I think that's when I began to think of her more as my daughter than my mother, on those nights when I heard her crying herself to sleep. From then on I cleaned the house, I walked the dog, I tried to warn her away from worthless men. By the time I was ten I often sat drinking tea with my no-nonsense Russian grandmother, both of us complaining about my mother as if she were a wild teenager and we were the irate guardians she regularly disobeyed.

It's possible that I became a writer because of my mother's fear of being alone after her divorce. A novelist, after all, is never alone. We travel with hundreds of people, invented characters that have already been written or will someday appear on the page. Despite my mother's uninhibited, untidy ways, she was the first heroine in my everyday life. She survived her failed marriage. She went onward, into the territory of single women and broken hearts. She fell in love again (wrong

man, wrong time, but love is always an act of courage).
She became a teacher and then a social worker, helping
hundreds of children in foster care, and she had a large
group of loving friends. She would rather see a play on
Broadway than clean the kitchen. She preferred taking
a class at The New School to cooking dinner. I thought
she was irresponsible. Most girls are angry with their
mothers at some point, and I was often furious with
mine. But the traits I once deplored are the ones I now
appreciate most. My mother possessed a true gift: she
had the ability to enjoy herself. She saw the beauty of
the world.

Perhaps that's the link that connects the women I
admire most. My grandmother Lillie, who volunteered
at an old-age home into her eighties, who lost a husband
and a child and still kept on going, one foot in front of
the other, out of Russia, across the ocean, to a tenement
in the Lower East Side of New York. She sold under-
wear and did alterations at a little shop she opened on
Jerome Avenue in the Bronx, where she kept a hammer
ready in the back room in case there were robbers. She

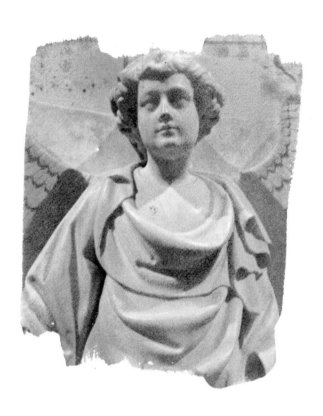

split her meager retirement check with me to help me become a writer. She was my angel, the person I could always depend on, as funny as she was tough. I spoke to her every morning until the day she died. Because of her, I know that if you are lucky enough to have one person believe in you, you have it made.

My sister-in-law Jo Ann was the bravest of the brave. She was eighteen when she fell in love with my brother. For a while she was a hippie in San Francisco. She worked in an incense factory, then she was a DJ at a radio station that operated out of a metal shack. She loved travel, painting, her children, and odd, interesting people. She had the best laugh in the world. When she was told she had only one more summer in which to live and was advised to attend to her bucket list, she informed the doctor she'd already done everything she'd ever wanted to do. Her life had been complete.

Again and again, friends have amazed me with their courage. My friend who lost her baby daughter at birth, and another who lost her child to an unexpected sudden illness, and still another who fights depression as if it were a dragon that follows her from town to town. A friend who battled cancer with extreme grace, not once but twice, a hairdresser who on her off hours helped women who had lost their hair, making them beautiful. She, herself, remained the same beautiful person she'd always been, with or without hair. You could take one look at her face and know she understood joy. In a last card to me she wrote: *Life is beautiful, just very unfair.*

My heroes don't give up, even when the going gets rough, even when they want to. They manage to see the stars in the sky until they disappear from sight, a glittering memory of our world.

"Hope" is the thing with feathers –
  That perches in the soul –
  And sings the tune without the words –
  And never stops – at all –

                    —Emily Dickinson

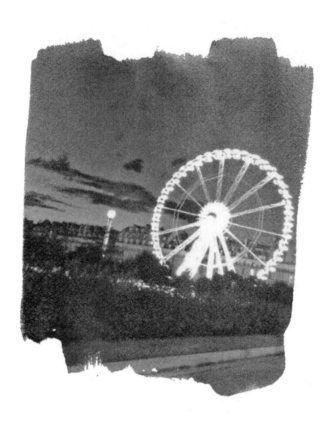

Choose
to Enjoy
Yourself

Start by eating chocolate. In fact, if you can, eat whatever you want. Any time. Any place. Cook your dream dinner: lasagna, stuffed mushrooms, fried rice, devil's food cake with mocha frosting, blueberry pie.

Take a cooking class. My son was in a class taught by the great Julia Child. He learned to make sublime eggs, poached, scrambled, coddled, and boiled. Here is the recipe for Julia's hard-boiled egg. It's simple, but most perfect things are.

Select a room-temperature egg.

Place in a pot of cold water.

Bring to a boil. When at a full boil, cover and remove the pot from the burner.

Let stand covered for fourteen minutes.

Submerge egg into ice-cold water. Peel.

I don't think Julia would mind me giving out her secret. She was a survivor. When we worked together raising funds at the hospital where we had both been treated, I instantly wished she was my best friend. Her warmth and compassion were legend. She didn't want to talk about herself and was deeply interested in other people. She knew who she was, but she didn't know who you were, and she wanted to. Frankly, she was more alive than people half her age. Everything was beautiful to her: an egg, a stranger's life story, a battered cooking pot.

Another secret recipe comes from my dear friend Maclin Bocock Guerard, who was a writer from Virginia and the most charming person I have ever known. She fell in love with her professor at Harvard, who was also my professor many years later, only she married him, which I would have, had I been in her shoes. Professor Guerard was the greatest writing teacher of his time; without him I would have never become a published writer. He was my mentor until the day he died, but Maclin was always my first reader. I trusted her completely. How often does that happen in a life? They were both beautiful and brilliant, and in spite of that they were also terribly kind.

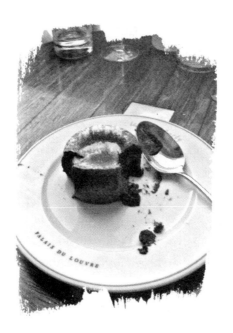

For my wedding present Maclin sent a double boiler and a recipe for brownies. I lost the double boiler, but I still have the recipe, typed out on an index card. No recipe comes close to this one. When you eat these brownies you will forget your sorrows. The sensation won't last, but it will be worth it. For a brief time, you will be in a chocolate ecstasy.

MACLIN'S BROWNIES

Melt 9 ounces of Nestle's semi-sweet chocolate bits over hot water (double boiler!) with 1 stick butter cut into pieces.

Beat 2 eggs with ½ cup white sugar until thick. Add ½ cup white flour, sifted with ¼ teaspoon salt and ½ teaspoon baking powder. Add the chocolate mixture and 1 teaspoon of vanilla and 1 cup (or less if you prefer) of walnut bits. Pour batter into 8" x 8" greased pan. Mix about 2 tablespoons of brown sugar with 1 teaspoon of melted butter and dot the top of the brownies. Bake at 375° for about 20 minutes, sometimes longer. Test with a toothpick. Cool on a rack after baking. When brownies have cooled, sprinkle with powdered sugar (you may use a doily set over brownies if you prefer a sugar pattern).

Here is a warning: Maclin's brownies will not appear to be perfect. They will sink in the middle. The top will crack. You'll want to throw them out. Don't. They will be everything they should be and more. They are perfect inside, which is even better than merely looking good. Soon you'll find yourself copying this recipe onto index cards to give to people you love, as Maclin did for me.

The last time I saw her, my friend was in the final stages of Parkinson's disease and could no longer speak. Her muscles would freeze and moving was difficult for her. We sat in her garden in Palo Alto. It was quiet and green and we could hear people playing tennis next door. We had already said everything we needed to in the letters we had written to each other for more than thirty years. All the same, I thanked her for the double boiler and for everything else she had given me.

Choose
Your
Friends

When you have a dinner party only invite people you want to talk to. Invite those you've always wanted to know. If I could, I would invite the Brontës and Edgar Allan Poe. They would be my first choices for dinner guests. I would want to know about their minds and his life. I would also want to invite Emily Dickinson, even though it is said that at some point she only spoke to callers through her bedroom door. That makes me love her all the more because I often feel exactly the same and want to hide away. She took to covering the windows in her bedroom, so she would feel safe, but she also went into the woods and collected hundreds of specimens of wildflowers.

Since it is impossible to invite great, dead writers, invite alive young people. Girls with pink hair who have big dreams. Young men who plan to change the world. Children who get into trouble at school because they have too much energy and too many ideas. People in the middle of their lives are so busy working, buying things, and trying to pay their mortgages that they often don't have time to spend dreaming out loud. Your friends' children may now seem more interesting than their parents. It may come as a complete surprise when they are the ones who take time to visit, who view you without judgment even though you have lost your hair and your eyebrows. They ask questions other people are too polite to bring up: Did you love her? Does it hurt? Are you afraid of what happens next?

I especially appreciated the fearlessness of teen readers and writers when I was undergoing treatment. One beautiful girl said to me, *I am the darkest person you've ever met,* but her poems were graceful and eloquent, and she hugged me when I left. Another told me that my book *Green Angel*—about a girl who loses everything and has to reclaim her life through writing her story—had gotten her through months in a hospital bed and several surgeries. I realized these teens were just starting out and I might be ending, but I felt a wild sort of joy to see how alike we were despite the difference in our ages. The fact that they loved books assured me that even if I wasn't able to be a part of it, the future would be in good hands.

I also found myself drawn to older people. I asked them, *How did it feel to see yourself change on the outside and look entirely different?* I began to talk to neighbors in their eighties and nineties, people who had previously been nothing more than nodding acquaintances. I discovered what interesting lives they'd led and how much they had to say. Once I slowed down and took the time to ask questions, I realized they had a thousand and one stories.

I threw a party for my mother's birthday, inviting both her friends and mine. We had tea in an old New England Inn. It was the last birthday my mother celebrated. We didn't know that, but we had an idea that might be true. We didn't count calories or glasses of wine. One of the younger women asked if there was anything the older women wished they'd done when they were younger and had more energy and time. The older women all agreed upon the answer: They wished they had traveled the world. But more importantly, they wished they'd fallen in love more often. *Don't hold back!* they told us. *Live right now!*

Make time for old friends. Get a group of your favorite people together and rent a room at a hotel. Order room service, watch movies, dance until the management starts to get complaints from other guests. Go to a spa together or make pizza from scratch. Tell someone how much he means to you. *Don't hold back!* Throw your arms around somebody right now.

The truth is, some of your closest friends may disappear during your most difficult times. These people have their own history and traumas; they may not be able to deal with yours. They may belong to the *before*.

I still mourn the loss of certain people, friends who didn't call after my diagnosis, who were too afraid to come to the hospital or visit me on my worst days. I was hurt. I felt abandoned. Looking back on it, I wish I had let them go more easily. If people aren't there for you now, when you really need them, they never will be, and it's time to move on. You'll be amazed by how many new friends you have in the *after*. They'll be the ones who aren't afraid of sorrow, who know we can't avoid it. The best we can do is face it together.

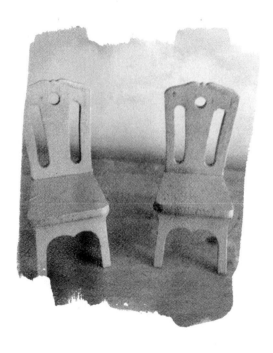

Choose
Whose Advice
You Take

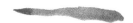

Take out your grandmother's letters and read them. In my opinion grandmothers know everything, although often when they're telling us what life is about, we think they're nagging us, or judging us, or trying to control us. Sooner or later, it sinks in. They've pretty much been right about everything. In each letter she sent, my grandmother's recommendations remained constant. *Don't take rides with strangers, don't drink soda, watch out for chemicals, don't forget to write. Listen to me and follow my advice. I won't mislead you. I am out only for your best interest and good health. You have sense. I put my hopes on you.*

When my brother and sister-in-law lived in San Francisco in the '70s, my grandmother, who considered them to be hippies, wrote, *They have no home, no job, no clothes, what does that prove? They look like they just stepped out of Siberia. I would not want to spend my youth that way. By the time they change, if they ever do, they will be older and then nothing is the same. Alice, listen to me. I am talking from experience. You only live once and that passes by fast.*

As it turns out my grandmother was wrong about my brother, who after living in a communal house in the Mission District went on to receive a PhD from MIT. She was also wrong about my sister-in-law, who became the mother of two wonderful sons who grew up to be everything my grandmother would have hoped they would be. But my grandmother was right about the most important point—time did pass fast, and when you are old nothing is the same. Are there people who realize what a gift youth is when they are in the midst of that shaggy, beautiful time of their lives? Probably not, but you finally do. So don't talk to boring people and don't take rides with strangers. But if you want to dress like you just walked out of Siberia, feel free to do so. Go to San Francisco. Wear flowers in your hair. But listen to my grandmother when she says you only live once.

As far as we know.

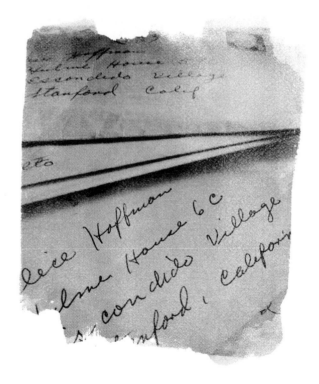

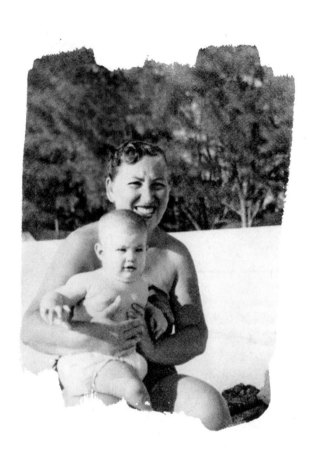

Choose
Your
Relatives

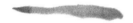

They say you can't choose your family. But you can choose the people you'll spend time with and who will receive cards notifying them you are currently unavailable. Relatives can be tricky when you are undergoing treatment for a disease or are in the throes of any sort of tragedy. Some want to do too much, some too little. But some are just right. A pie left on your back porch is just right. A hug in the hallway. A book of poems sent through the mail.

Only answer the phone when you want to, and then, give yourself permission to say you can't talk, especially if it's a relative. Make up an excuse. *There's someone at my door, a bear is in the living room, there's a meteor shower spilling over my front lawn.* Or just tell the truth. *I'm tired. I'm sick. I'm at a loss. I'm not ready to talk. Call me later, tomorrow, next month. Better still, let me call you back.*

I learned from my mistakes. I didn't experience illness in my family until Jo Ann was diagnosed with brain cancer. For some reason I thought life always got better, but it was nearly a full year of things getting worse. When she was failing there was an afternoon when we sat together and she told me she was afraid to die. I quickly said, *Don't be silly, that's not going to happen.* The words were out of my mouth before I had time to think. But it was happening, as it does to all of us, only she was dying sooner rather than later and she knew it. She had been very brave and had sworn she would make history. When doctors found a cure, she would be on the cover of *Time* magazine. That's what she had hoped for, but that's not how it turned out.

I was with her every day of her illness, but at the

very end, I had plans to take my children on vacation. I waivered and thought I should stay, but Jo Ann said to me, *Go! And don't feel guilty!*

She knew exactly what I needed to hear. Those were the last words she ever said to me. She died while I was in the desert in Arizona with my husband and children. She allowed me to understand I'd done everything I could for her, and that I, and everyone who loved her, had to step away and go on living.

Now I know what she wanted from me on the day she told me she was afraid. It was exactly what I wanted when I had cancer and I thought I was going to die. I should have sat down next to her, put my arms around her, and told her that I loved her. That's all anyone wants. It took me a long time to figure this out. It's a complicated human puzzle. But it's never too late to know that love is all you need.

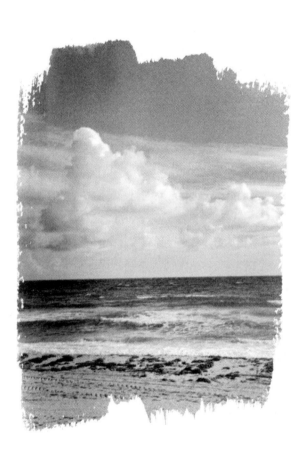

Choose
How You Spend
Your Time

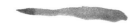

Watch every old movie you've always wanted to see. Fall in love with Clark Gable. Watch comedies that involve bridesmaids, pretty women, men at bachelor parties, teenagers and hot tubs, and anything with Bill Murray. I highly recommend the original *Wuthering Heights*, even though it is a strange mash-up of the first and second halves of the book. Laurence Olivier is worth it. Who wouldn't fall in love with him? Two more words that need no explanation: Johnny Depp.

Don't watch movies about cancer. Avoid anything focusing on death, sorrow, or illness. Sometimes these themes sneak up on you. You think you're watching a comedy when suddenly a major character will need to undergo chemotherapy or be wheeled into the ER. Interestingly enough, they'll still look great. Under certain circumstances, no one looks great. Oh sure, they can look attractive, even if they are wearing a head scarf or weeping in a hospital, but no one looks movie-star great.

You may want to pick a day when you watch every tearjerker ever made, starting with *Tender Mercies*. Sometimes it feels good just to cry. If you do this, make sure you have tissues and a big batch of Maclin's brownies.

Don't forget books. What would life be without them? Emily Brontë, Edgar Allan Poe, F. Scott Fitzgerald, Toni Morrison, Jane Austen, William Faulkner. Read the greats—they're great for a reason. They know how to chart the human soul.

Revisit the stories you loved as a child—you'll love

them even more now. Start with Andrew Lang's fairy books, books sorted by color. *Red, Lilac,* and *Blue* are my favorites. Sometimes I think we can learn everything we need to know about the world when we read fairy tales. *Be careful, be fearless, be honest, leave a trail of crumbs to lead you home again.*

In a novel, you'll find yourself in a world of possibilities. You'll find shelter there. I spent one entire summer reading Ray Bradbury. I was twelve, which can be a terrible year. It's the summer when you suddenly know you will never be a child again. Being an adult may not look so good. The world that awaits you is scary and huge. This is when you want to stop time, be a kid, ride your bike. But everyone around you is growing up, and you have to, too.

I remained in Ray Bradbury's world for as long as possible. It was a place where it was possible to recognize good from evil, darkness from light. I was a cynical kid, and I didn't have much faith in the world, but I trusted Ray Bradbury. I took everything he said personally. Often I would read until the fireflies came out.

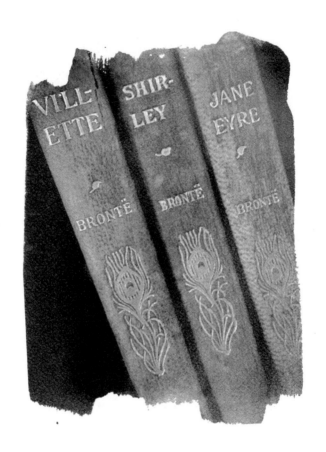

I read because I wanted to escape sadness, which was a big theme in my family. My great-grandfather had been forced into the czar's army, where he served for twenty years, before he shot off his toes with a rifle so they would finally let him go. Because we were Russian, sadness came naturally to us. But so did reading. In my family, a book was a life raft.

I've often wondered if I spent too much time inside of books. If perhaps I ended up getting lost in there. I feared that reading, and later writing, stopped me from living a full life in the real world. I still don't know the answer to this, but I'm not sure I would have gotten past being twelve without Ray Bradbury, and I know that imagining the plot for my novel *The River King* during a lengthy bone scan helped me get through that test. The hospital faded and I was walking through a small town where I knew everyone. I slipped into the river, past the water lilies, past the muddy shore. Here was my life raft. A book.

When the technician told me the test was over, I was amazed, thinking we had just begun. But three hours had already passed. I'd been gone all that time. I'd been in another world entirely.

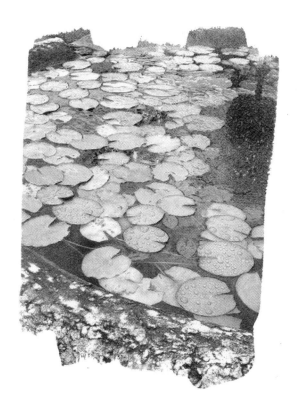

Choose
to Plan for
the Future

Write your troubles on a slip of paper and burn it.

Now make a list of what you want to do next year.

My plan was to pack a bag and head for Cape Cod. When I imagined going there, I could taste the blueberries that grew at the edge of the woods. I could see blackbirds in the trees, lily pads in the pond, sea lavender in the marsh.

Your favorite beach town will be waiting for you next year. As the darkness sifts down, you will catch fireflies in a glass. You will go to brunch every morning even if it isn't Sunday and order French toast, even though you swore off carbohydrates five years ago. Imagine yourself on a screened-in porch next summer, drinking iced tea. Collect shells, fall in love, read ten novels in a row.

In October you'll see the leaves change. Collect the ones in the shape of stars, go to Vermont, buy maple syrup and pots of chrysanthemums. When December arrives, you'll take your mother or your niece to see the Rockettes in the Radio City Christmas Spectacular. You'll watch snow fall in Paris or in your hometown. Make a list, check it twice, you still have plenty to do.

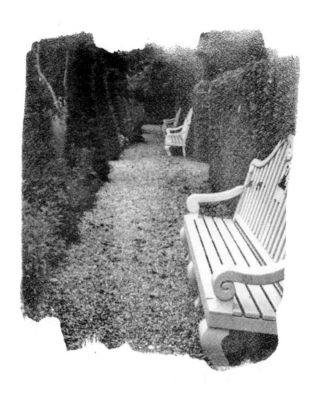

The woods are lovely, dark, and deep,

But I have promises to keep,

And miles to go before I sleep,

And miles to go before I sleep.

—Robert Frost

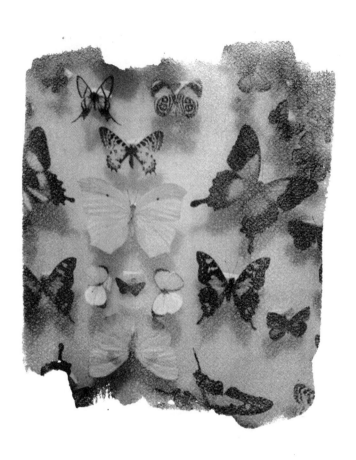

Choose to
Love
Who You Are

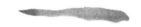

You will get old, fat, thin. You'll look sad, tired, worn-out, dragged down, bummed out. So what? You'll still have the same killer smile, your one-of-a-kind laugh, those eyes.

Eyes say everything—they show what's inside you whether you're six or ninety-six. I remember my grandmother telling me she was shocked every time she passed a mirror. She expected to see a beautiful sixteen-year-old girl, and instead she saw an old woman. But she was still sixteen when she laughed. And when I looked in her eyes I knew exactly who she was.

Don't judge yourself harshly. Don't listen to people who do. Some changes are temporary, though they seem like forever. People say whoever discovers the cure for baldness brought on by chemotherapy will win a Nobel Prize. I agree. When this time comes, women with cancer will grow their hair long just because they can. They'll wear braids, waves, bangs; they'll use hair dye in shades of red that attract bees and young men. Eyebrows will remain in place, like beautiful black butterflies, and children will not be frightened of baldness, because it will have lost its meaning. Bald woman will likely become a fad when this happens, filling up fashion magazines with beautiful, pouty baldness so that at long last we realize that being bald only serves to point out a person's most beautiful features.

Choose
to Accept
Sorrow

D uring my radiation treatment I read *Man's Search for Meaning*. People said, *Isn't that book depressing?* But it wasn't. It was honest. The author, Viktor Frankl, was a psychiatrist who lost nearly everyone he loved in the Holocaust. This fact already makes your problems feel small even if you are in the radiation waiting room. Frankl later developed a theory about tragedy and sorrow, that it is these experiences that make us human and define who we are.

I was looking for an answer in the waiting room. It was the beginning of my search for advice on how to survive. Here is the lesson I learned from Frankl about his time in a concentration camp, an explanation of how certain people were able to continue on despite extreme darkness:

We had to learn ourselves and, furthermore, we had to teach the despairing men, that it did not really matter what we expected from life, but rather what life expected from us. We needed to stop asking about the meaning of life, and instead to think of ourselves as those who were being questioned by life—daily and hourly. Our answer must consist, not in talk and meditation, but in right action and in right conduct. Life ultimately means taking the responsibility to find the right answer to its problems and to fulfill the task which it constantly sets for each individual.

We are all responsible for our actions, and our reactions. We are responsible for how we respond to situations we cannot control. I could not run away from my circumstances, or control the path of my disease, but I could control what I did with my experience of that illness. I chose to become a fund-raiser for breast cancer. That was the right answer to my problem. As a matter of fact, I think it may be the rightest and best answer I've ever found. When you help others, your own troubles aren't as heavy. In fact, you can fold them like a handkerchief and place them in your pocket. They're still there, but they're not the only thing you carry.

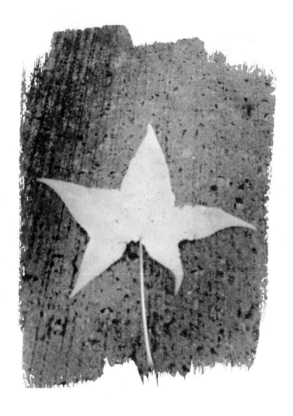

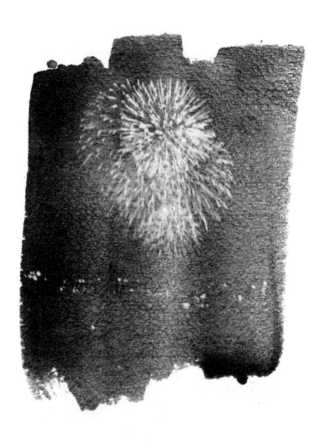

Choose
to Dream

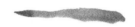

Plan the trip you always wanted to take. You didn't have time before, you couldn't afford it, you were afraid to fly. Now just buy the ticket and stop thinking so much. You'll pay it off later. You'll take a Valium. Now you know that you have to make time.

Buy guidebooks, walking shoes, maps, a beautiful sweater that you think you can't afford. There is Barcelona, there is your hometown, there is an inn right down the street. If you have no dream destination, take mine—Venice. Stay at a hotel on the Grand Canal. I stayed at the Danieli Hotel in the room where the writer George Sand had a love affair with Frédéric Chopin. It was a small, beautiful room. Amazing that so much passion could be contained in that room, number ten, the most requested room in the hotel, though there are far larger and more beautiful suites.

I thought of all the people who had fallen in love over the centuries within the same walls. The key to the room was kept on a red silk string. I believe Chopin held this same key. Above the door, the names of the most famous of those lovers is written on the wall. If I had one day to live over and over again, it would be that one.

Walk through the St. Mark's Square at night in the fog, take a speedboat to the Lido beach, eat pasta, shrimp, and gelato. In a gondola you will remember a day you had radiation, or the day you lost your mother, or the scar you will always carry with you. You may start to cry. Your tears will fall into the Grand Canal as you pass by the Basilica di San Marco. For that moment you will remember everything you have been through and all that lies ahead of you in your life. It's not easy. It never is. That is the secret our parents fail to tell us, out of kindness and love, but it's a secret we need to know. Everything that begins, ends. Everything beautiful disappears. You'll know this as you watch hail fall and disappear into puddles on the plaza. The canals will change color from blue to green to gray and then, at last, the sky will clear. Even when these things disappear, when they're over and done and you are back home, you will remember it all, including the day you stood before the Bridge of Sighs.

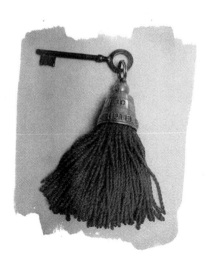

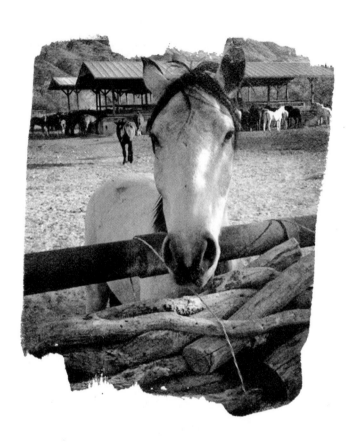

Choose
Something
New

Do those things you always wanted to do but never tried because you thought you would fail. You were certain you didn't have the talent, or the time, or the energy. Take up knitting, bird watching, or yoga. Take charge of a chore you've been putting off. Clean your closet, and bring all of your old clothes to a shelter. You may see women there who will break your heart. When they put on your clothes, they will look like you, just a you who took a wrong turn. Every woman is only one bad boyfriend or one bad choice away from the street. And she's only one good choice back to the path that will lead her home.

If you try and fail at some new endeavor, what difference does it make? None at all, unless you are jumping out of a plane. But when it comes to most skills, failure is the only way to become better at something. Knitting teaches you that. You may have to unwind all of your stitches and start anew. That doesn't mean you've wasted your time. You learn from every stitch, even those that don't amount to anything. All writers should be made to knit a hat before they start writing a novel. It would help with understanding the importance of revision, and that the process is what can bring you the most joy.

Here is a wonderful hat pattern created by my cousin Lisa, who once knitted a wedding dress for *Vogue Knitting*. You can knit in a waiting room, a car, a funeral parlor, anywhere at all. You can knit for yourself, for someone you just met, or for a person you love dearly.

Bald people are especially grateful for this gift.

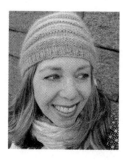

BEEHIVE HAT

by Lisa Hoffman

Level: Beginner / Intermediate

Materials:

DK weight 100% merino wool or alternative yarn
(approx 175 yds / 160 m).

To work flat: One size 6 (4.0 mm) straight or
24" circular needle.

To work in the round: One 16" size 6 (4.0 mm)
circular needle; one set size 6 (4.0 mm) double
point needles; marker.

Tapestry needle for seaming and darning ends.

Size: Adult Small / Med (hat can be made larger or
smaller by adding or removing stitches in multiples of 8).

Gauge: 20 sts and 26 rows = 4" in Stockinette Stitch; adjust needle size if necessary to obtain correct gauge.

Stitch Guide:

Knit 1, Purl 1 Ribbing (A) (work flat—multiples of 2)

Row 1 (RS): *K1, p1; rep from * to last stitch, k1.

Row 2 (WS): *P1, k1; rep from * to last stitch, p1.

Repeat rows 1 and 2 for pattern.

Knit 1, Purl 1 Ribbing (B) (worked in the round— multiples of 2)

Round 1: *K1, p1; repeat from * to end of round.

Repeat round 1 for pattern.

Stockinette Stitch

Row 1 (RS): Knit.

Row 2 (WS): Purl.

Repeat rows 1 and 2 for pattern.

Reverse Stockinette Stitch

Row 1 (RS): Purl.

Row 2 (WS): Knit.

Repeat rows 1 and 2 for pattern.

Note: When working in rounds, knitting every round creates Stockinette Stitch and purling every round creates Reverse Stockinette Stitch.

Abbreviations:

K2tog: Knit 2 together

Rev St st: Reverse Stockinette Stitch

St st: Stockinette Stitch

RS: Right side

WS: Wrong side

. . . .

Hat *(knit flat)*

Cast on 98 sts. Work Knit 1, Purl 1 Ribbing (A) for
6 rows. Change to work body of hat as follows:

Rows 1–6: Rev St st (purl on right side, knit on wrong
side).

Rows 7–12: St st (knit on right side, purl on wrong side).

Repeat rows 1–12 three times more, then rows 1–6 once
more.

Work 2 rows St st. Begin crown decreases as follows:

Row 1 (RS): Knit 1, *knit 6, k2tog, repeat from * to last
stitch, knit 1.

Row 2: Purl.

Row 3: Knit 1, *knit 5, k2tog, repeat from * to last stitch,
knit 1.

Row 4: Purl.

Row 5: Knit 1, *knit 4, k2tog, repeat from * to last stitch,
knit 1.

Row 6: Purl.

Continue to decrease in this manner, working one less stitch before decrease every other row as established until 14 stitches remain.

Next row (RS): Knit 1, *knit 2, k2tog, repeat from * 3 times, end knit 1. Eleven stitches remain.

Work 6 rows St st. Cut yarn leaving 12" and pull through remaining stitches. Seam hat, darn ends.

. . . .

Hat *(knit in the round)*

With 16" circular needle, cast on 96 sts. Join to work in rounds, being careful not to twist. Place marker to note end of round. Work Knit 1, Purl 1 Ribbing (B) for 6 rounds, slipping marker every round throughout pattern. Change to work body of hat as follows:

Rounds 1–6: Purl.

Rounds 7–12: Knit.

Repeat rounds 1–12 three times more, then rounds 1–6 once more. Knit 2 rounds.

Begin crown decreases as follows, changing to double pointed needles when stitches can no longer be worked comfortably on circular needle:

*Knit 6, k2tog, repeat from * to end of round.

Knit 1 round even.

*Knit 5, k2tog, repeat from * to end of round.

Knit 1 round even.

*Knit 4, k2tog, repeat from * to end of round.

Knit 1 round even.

Continue to decrease in this manner, working one less stitch before decrease every other round as established until 12 stitches remain.

Next round: *K2, k2tog, repeat from * 3 times. Nine stitches remain. Knit 6 rounds on these 9 stitches. Cut yarn and pull through remaining stitches.

Darn ends.

I know why my grandmother always told me to bring along a sweater on cold nights. She was telling me I had to take care of myself, to watch out for chills and pneumonia. But she was also telling me that life is worth fighting for. I have every blanket she ever made for me even though they are as heavy as armor. My grandmother's spirit is in every stitch, and her love for me is there as well.

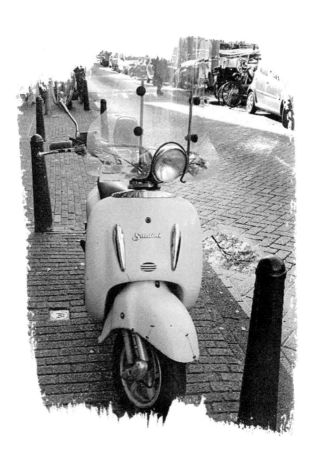

Choose to
Give In
to Yourself

Take a nap whenever you want to. Look at the tree outside your window for an hour without being ashamed that you might be wasting time.

Go and don't feel guilty.

Time is different now. Don't worry about wasting it. It belongs to you. There are programs on television that will surprise you, things you never paid attention to before when you were so busy and never took time for yourself. You may get caught up in trashy dramas about high school passions or become obsessed with a reality show about fishermen or storage units.

Play music. Listen to Sheryl Crow, Lady Gaga, Bruce Springsteen, Van Morrison. Remember where you were when you first heard your favorite songs and who you were in love with back then. I remember where I was when I first heard the Beatles, Bob Dylan, Judy Collins, Mick Jagger. *Who knows where the time goes?* The music of your youth stays with you and winds itself around your heart. I hear one chord of "Strawberry Fields Forever" or "Satisfaction" and am instantly back in time. It doesn't matter where I am, suddenly I'm walking through the woods, I'm in my best friend's room plotting how we might run off to London (never happened); I'm with my mother standing outside The Plaza Hotel, screaming every time a curtain moves because Paul McCartney might be there.

In the middle of a crisis, you may decide to get a puppy. People will tell you you're crazy. This is the worst time to make a life change. In some instances this is correct: trauma and major decisions should probably not go hand and hand. Most people agree that someone undergoing treatment for a serious disease or

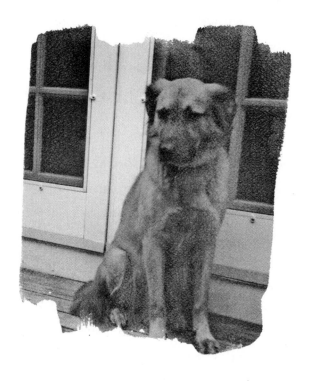

experiencing great loss should put off getting a divorce or ending a lifelong friendship. But a puppy is never a mistake, though it is often a mess.

Make sure you have backup—someone who can take it for walks on days when you can't, or, let's be honest, someone willing to adopt your puppy if your circumstances change. Everyone needs backup, a friend you can count on, a sister you argue with every time you see her, but would trust with your life. Everyone needs a plan B, especially when there's a creature that depends on you.

My puppy came in a crate from Syracuse plastered with stickers that read, *I'm a puppy, be nice to me.* He was a Polish Sheepdog who sat in the window above the couch where I spent a great deal of time during the months of my chemo treatment. He got so big he had to squash himself into the space between the couch and the window ledge. He watched the leaves with me. He became a leaf expert, and so did I. We both decided nothing was more beautiful or more interesting. I never felt alone when I was with him. Sometimes that's what you need most of all, not to be alone. Sometimes a dog knows that before you do.

Time has passed and my sheepdog is now blind. He has difficulty getting onto the couch. But I still think he can make out the shapes of falling leaves.

Choose
to Make Things
Beautiful

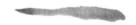

P eople say no man on his deathbed ever said
he wished he spent more time at the office.
I disagree. I assume Pablo Picasso would
have said exactly that. Jane Austen would have agreed.
When your work brings you joy, you cannot get enough
of it. People who turn to work during times of trauma
aren't necessarily workaholics; they're in love with what
they do. In fairy tales, the pure of heart can spin straw
into gold; they take the stuff of everyday life and forge
it into something precious and lasting.

If you don't feel this way about your current work,

take the time to make something beautiful. Do it on a Saturday morning when everyone is asleep. Take out crayons, glitter, a camera, a notebook. Take a deep breath, then begin.

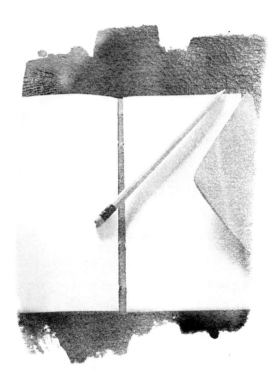

Choose
to Tell Your
Own Story

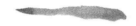

You can tell it however you want. It's your story.

I kept my illness a secret, sharing my diagnosis with only my closest friends and family. I'm still not sure why I did this, but it seems to me now it was a survival technique. For other people, telling everyone may work. I needed to process my issues on my own.

It's a good idea to sit down with your children and tell them what they mean to you. The saddest girl I ever knew wasn't told that her mother had cancer. Her mother just disappeared day one and came back different, and after that my friend was different, too. Every year some part of her disappeared. She stopped confiding in me. She didn't laugh the way she used to. After a while she wasn't my friend anymore.

Explain that because you are ill or sad you may be grumpy, sleepy, dopey, and all of the other things the dwarves in *Snow White* are. Assure your children you will still be available to watch mindless TV shows, eat M&Ms, and lose at board games. If you feel up to it, take them on a trip to an amusement park, or a beach, or the American Museum of Natural History. Sometimes children forget trips such as these, but these outings may make an indelible impression, and perhaps more importantly, you will always remember. When people ask about your terrible year, the first thing that will come to mind is the grin on your son's face on the roller coaster and how fast your daughter ran on the beach. She was almost flying. She was the most beautiful thing on earth.

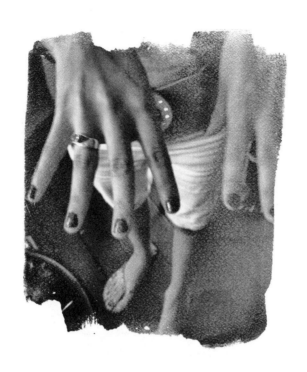

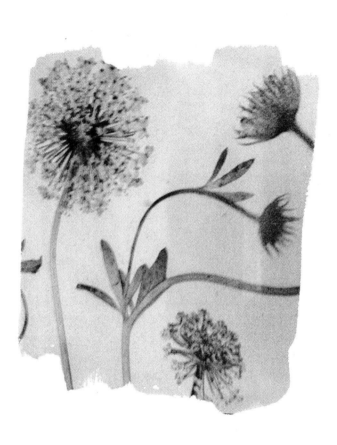

Choose
to Forgive

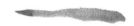

S tart with your mother, your sister, your ex–
best friend, the boss who fired you. Don't
hold grudges; it takes up too much energy.
Send postcards to these people. Write *good-bye* or *good
luck* or *good riddance*. Apologize to people you've wronged.
It will feel so good, you'll wonder why you waited this
long.

While I was undergoing treatment, I had lunch with
my father, something we hadn't done for years. He was
aging and I was ill; it was definitely time for me to
forgive him for never being there for me. I wanted to

say, *I understand, we all make mistakes,* but I couldn't get those words out. When my father apologized for being a terrible parent I wish I could have told him I had forgiven him, but my throat closed up and that was that. I hope he knew that I forgave him. It happened the moment he apologized.

If you can forgive someone, I highly recommend that you do. It will be like losing twenty pounds. Maybe even two hundred and twenty pounds.

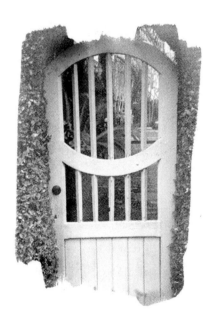

Choose to
Claim Your Past

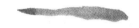

Visit your great aunt, your high school teacher in a rest home, the uncle who knows all of the secrets in your family. Collect family photographs and stories.

Videotape your aged aunt who doesn't know the current date but remembers the details of her girlhood in New Jersey. Interview your mother and you'll be amazed by what you discover. You used to wonder why older people sat together discussing illness and cures, and now you know the reason why. If you listen when various diseases are discussed you'll learn about varicose veins, the need for physical therapy, why acupuncturists are worth going to, how hot water and lemon in the morning is better for your health than coffee or tea. All of this is beginning to make sense.

Getting old is starting to look good to you now.

Buy a journal, a diary, a beautiful leather book. Write down the names of those who hurt you and those who helped you. Visit the house where you grew up and take photographs. Take out the dress you were married in, the sneakers you used to wear to high school, your mother's diamond ring. Make a time line. Use stickers, rubber stamps, everything you can to mark the best days of your life.

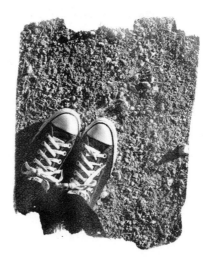

Choose
to Be
Yourself

Go get a tattoo if you always wanted one. A star, a dragon, your children's initials, Tinker Bell with pale green wings. Stay in your pajamas for days. Buy a pair of kick-ass boots. Go to a club and hear jazz, or drive to Cleveland to visit the Rock and Roll Hall of Fame. Start wearing red lipstick. Duck out of work and catch a Red Sox or a Yankees game, depending on where your loyalties lie. Order a margarita at four in the afternoon. Volunteer at the museum and be alone with the Egyptian artifacts early in the morning before anyone else has arrived. How is it possible that something made so long ago is still so beautiful? Gold, stone, turquoise, all of these elements have outlasted their owners. But all were made by hand.

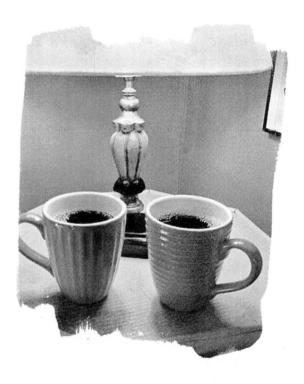

Choose
to Share

Talk to a stranger. Join a support group. Reach out even if you're not the sort of person who does that. Even if it's not your style.

When you share something, the act of sharing changes you. I remember calling friends of friends, people who were complete strangers to me, just to hear the story of their survivorship. In each case these women talked to me for hours. Though we had never met, they gave me their wisdom and shared their experiences. They had already been through the war and could report back as survivors who knew the score.

During my treatment for breast cancer I joined a support group. I am shy and usually unable to have a decent conversation with someone new, which means anyone I have known for less than twenty years. All the same, I found myself telling women who were complete strangers the most personal details of my life. We discussed night sweats and nightmares. Love, betrayal, fears, all of it, as if we had known one another not for twenty years, but a hundred and twenty.

If you join a support group, call one of these strangers in the middle of the night and cry. Go ahead; she won't be annoyed even if it's two in the morning. Unlike everyone else you know, she won't tell you everything is fine. She'll listen to you and she'll understand. Then she'll tell you you had better plan to survive.

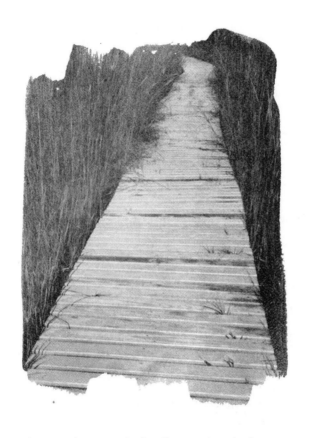

There's a long road of suffering ahead of you.
But don't lose courage . . . Help one another.
It is the only way to survive.

—Eli Wiesel, *Night*

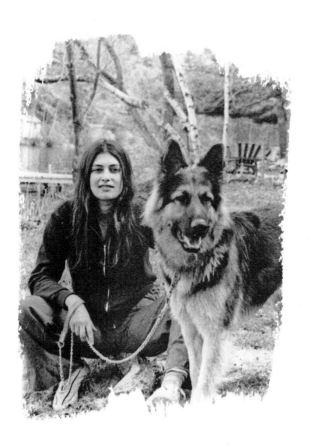

Choose
Love

You may feel alone, but your husband, lover, girlfriend, or wife is going through this with you. True, they are not the ones with needles in their arms or surgeries to recover from, but they have to watch you go through these things. Which is worse: to be the person who is ill, or the one who has to watch someone he loves suffer?

Both are not too good.

Sometimes the people who love you will be in denial. They can be rude and thoughtless. They may eat pizza in front of you when you are nauseated from chemo. They may miss appointments or say things like, *Why are you crying?* Responses like this may make you want to walk out the door. Sit beside them instead and hold their hand. Love is complicated, love can be hidden, love, above all else, is loyalty.

I sometimes say my first husband was a German shepherd, which in a way is true. I grew up with dogs, but Houdini was the first dog that belonged to me completely. We met on a farm in California. I fell for him instantly and brought him home without asking my roommates. He trained himself, and the truth of it is, he trained me. I would take him to class with me when I was a graduate student and he would sleep beneath my chair. Later, when I taught, he would sometimes pass gas from his spot beneath my chair. I didn't know if it would be even more embarrassing to assure the class that it was not me, so I just smiled and said nothing.

When I moved to New York City, I put on sunglasses and took Houdini to restaurants and to the old Elgin Theater on Eighth Avenue. I suppose people thought he was a guide dog when I brought him onto buses and trains, and he was exactly that for me. When we were in the woods he once came nose to nose with a baby deer. Toddlers and cats crawled over him and he remained serene. He taught me how to love someone. He lived for sixteen years. I continue to miss him every day, though I have had many other wonderful dogs since, and another husband, who is human and very nice and who went with me to every radiation and chemo visit.

My expectations of what I wanted in a man I learned from a dog: loyalty and kindness.

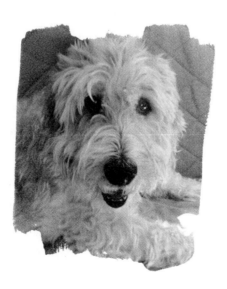

Choose
the Evidence

W rite it down. Even if it's a few sentences. Because you won't remember. You think you will never forget, but you will. Write down your life story or a poem. Sometimes shorter is better. Make a list of what all you have loved in this unfair and beautiful world. *Fireflies. Blue herons. Fresh coffee. Manhattan at dusk. The man waiting in the other room. The woman with dark eyes.*

When I couldn't write about characters that didn't have cancer and worried I might never get past this single experience, my oncologist told me that cancer didn't have to be my entire novel. It was just a chapter.

She assured me that eventually it wouldn't be the main character who had cancer, it would be the grandmother, then the best friend, then the distant cousin, the neighbor, and finally the stranger down the block. Your sorrow will become smaller, like a star in the daylight that you can't even see. It's there, shining, but there is also a vast expanse of blue sky.

All the same, some things stay with you forever. You are a different person now. You know it and I know it. You're not the same. You're a survivor. Congratulations.

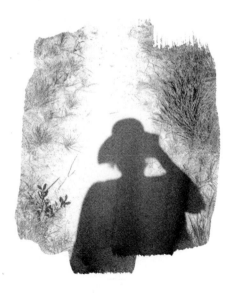